ALL I CAN HANDLE: I'm No Mother Teresa

A Life Raising Three Daughters with Autism

Kim Stagliano

Foreword by Jenny McCarthy

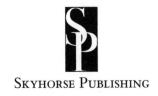

SKYHORSE PUBLISHING

Skyhorse Publishing books may be purchased in bulk at special discounts for sales promotion, corporate gifts, fund-raising, or educational purposes. Special editions can also be created to specifications.

For details, contact the Special Sales Department, Skyhorse Publishing, 555 Eighth Avenue, Suite 903, New York, NY 10018 or info@skyhorsepublishing.com.

www.skyhorsepublishing.com

10 9 8 7 6 5 4 3 2 1

Library of Congress Cataloging-in-Publication Data

Stagliano, Kim.
All I can handle-- I'm no Mother Teresa : a life raising three daughters with autism / Kim Stagliano.
p. cm.
ISBN 978-1-61608-069-3 (hardcover : alk. paper)
1. Stagliano, Kim. 2. Autistic children--Family relationships--United States. 3. Mothers of children with disabilities--United States--Biography. 4. Mothers and daughters. I. Title.
RJ506.A9S724 2010
618.92'858820092--dc22
[B]
2010022011

Printed in the United States of America